HUMAN FACE
ANATOMY COLORING BOOK

Facial Anatomy Coloring Workbook for Injectors and Medical Students

WITH COMPLETE SOLUTIONS

THIS BOOK
BELONGS TO:

_____

_____

_____

Facial Muscles - *Frontal view*

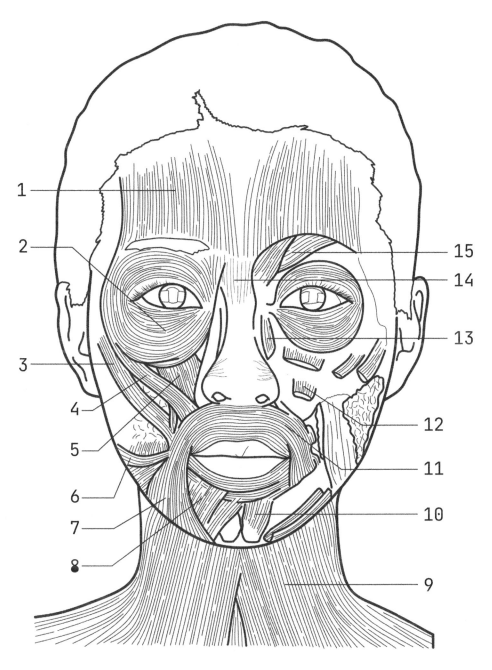

1	_____	9	_____
2	_____	10	_____
3	_____	11	_____
4	_____	12	_____
5	_____	13	_____
6	_____	14	_____
7	_____	15	_____
8	_____		

Facial Muscles - *Oblique View*

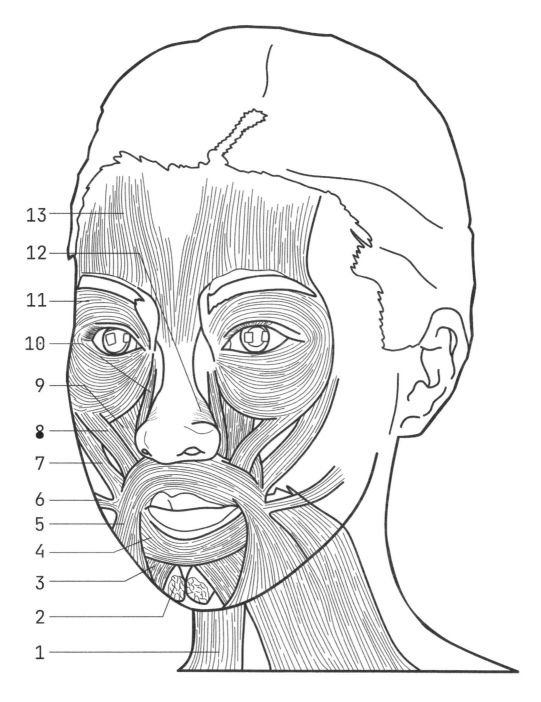

1 _____   8 _____

2 _____   9 _____

3 _____   10 _____

4 _____   11 _____

5 _____   12 _____

6 _____   13 _____

7 _____

Facial Muscles - *Lateral View*

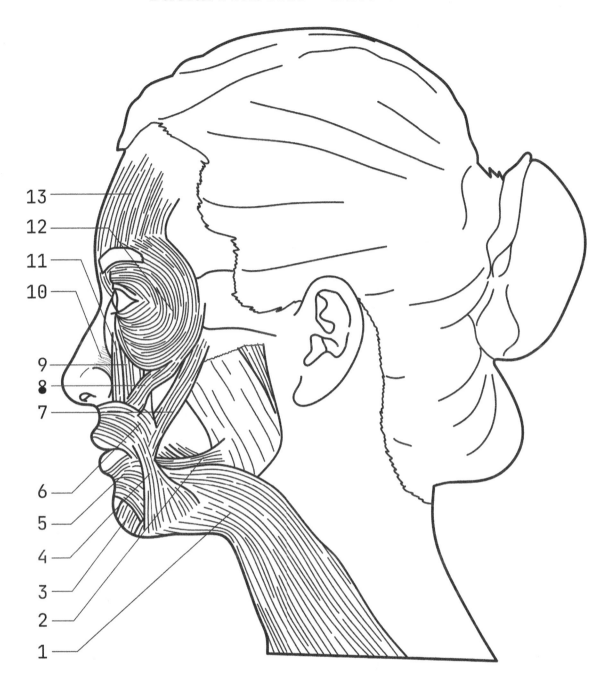

1 _____   8 _____

2 _____   9 _____

3 _____   10 _____

4 _____   11 _____

5 _____   12 _____

6 _____   13 _____

7 _____

Muscles of the Lower Face

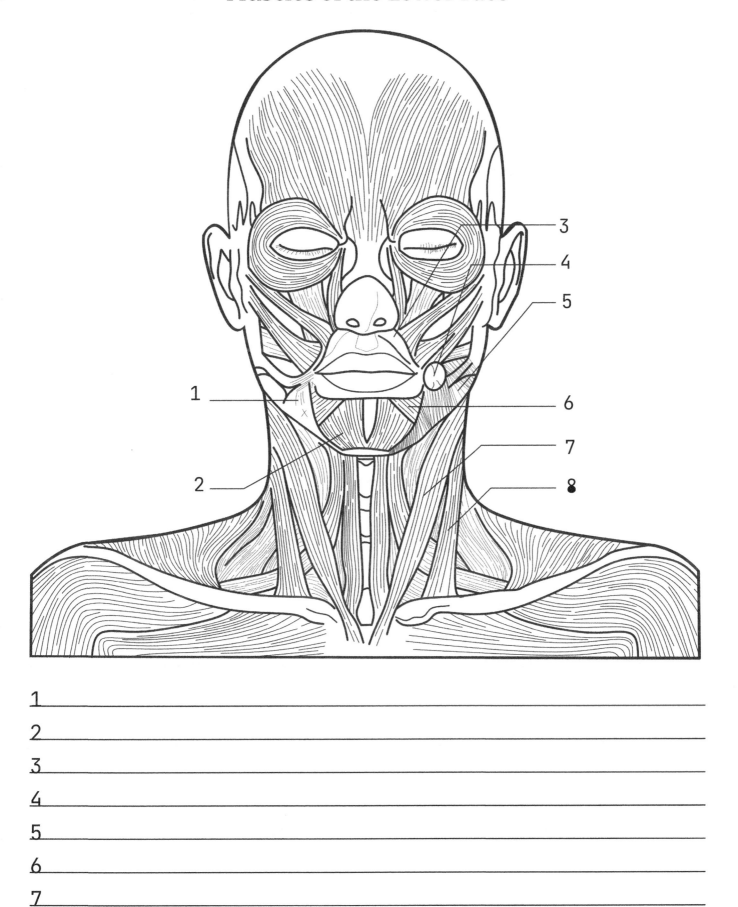

1 _____
2 _____
3 _____
4 _____
5 _____
6 _____
7 _____
8 _____

Muscles of the Midface

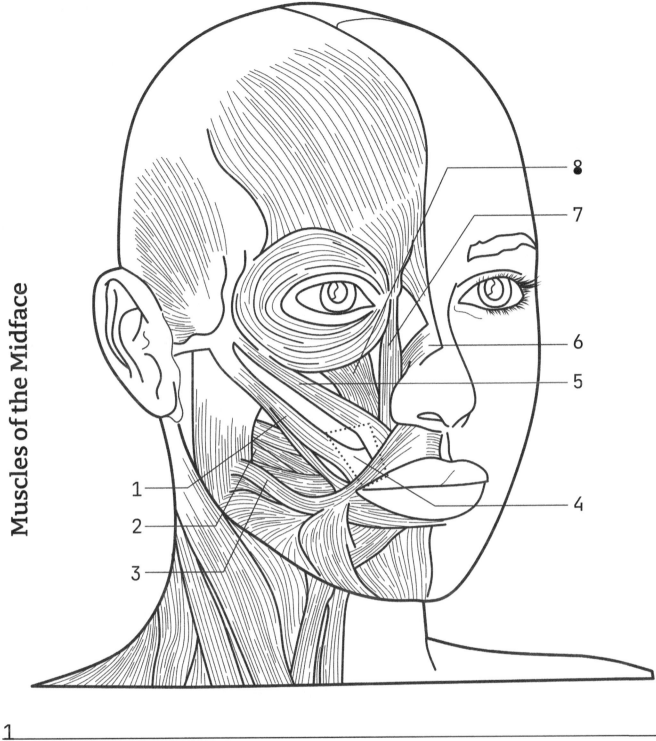

8

7

6

5

4

1

2

3

1 _____

2 _____

3 _____

4 _____

5 _____

6 _____

7 _____

8 _____

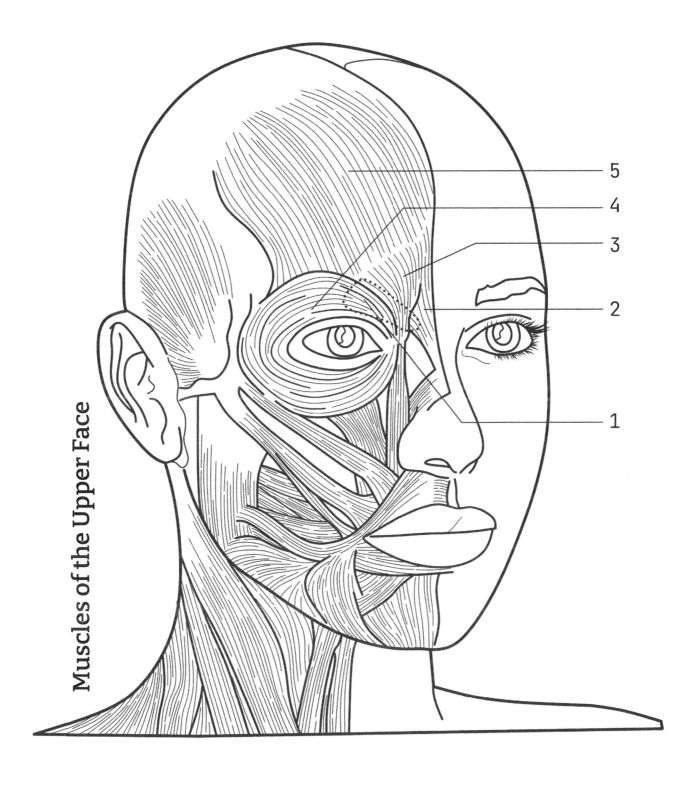

Muscles of the Upper Face

5

4

3

2

1

1 _____

2 _____

3 _____

4 _____

5 _____

Perinasal Muscles

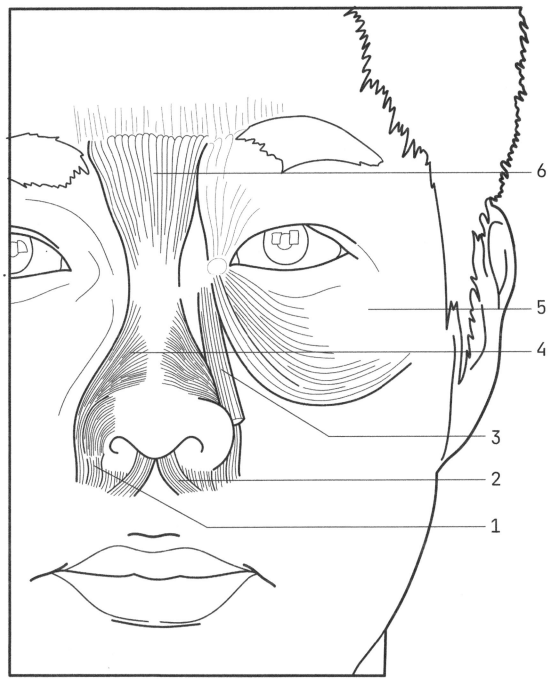

1 _____

2 _____

3 _____

4 _____

5 _____

6 _____

Perioral Muscles

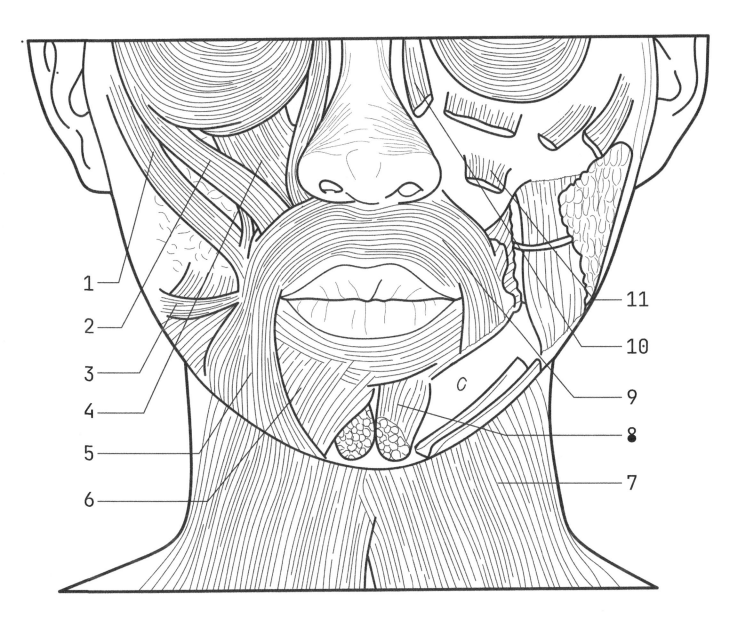

1 _____   7 _____

2 _____   8 _____

3 _____   9 _____

4 _____   10 _____

5 _____   11 _____

6 _____

Superficial Perioral Muscles

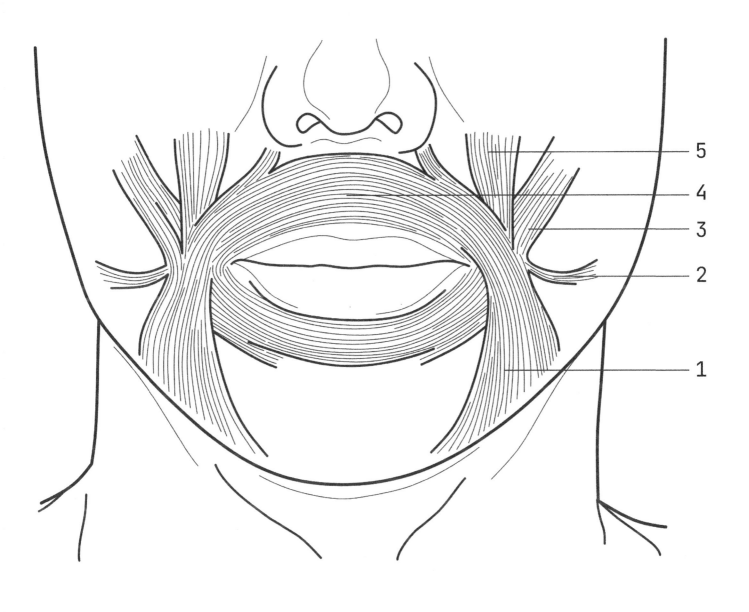

5 _____

4 _____

3 _____

2 _____

1 _____

1 _____

2 _____

3 _____

4 _____

5 _____

Anatomical Layers of the Face - *Basic Five Layers of the Face*

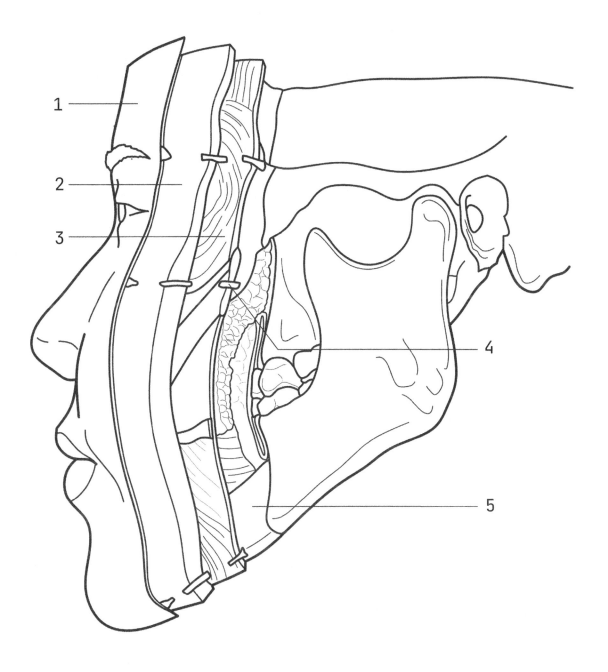

1 _____

2 _____

3 _____

4 _____

5 _____

Anatomical Layers of the Forehead and Glabella

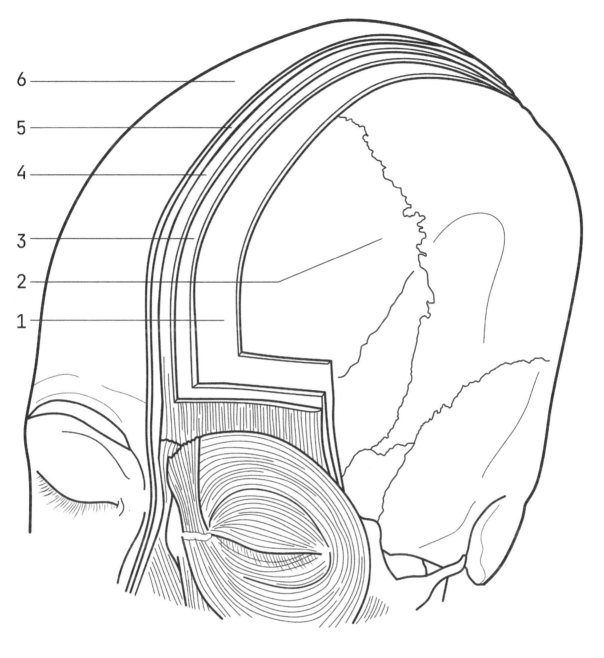

6 _____

5 _____

4 _____

3 _____

2 _____

1 _____

Arteries of the Face

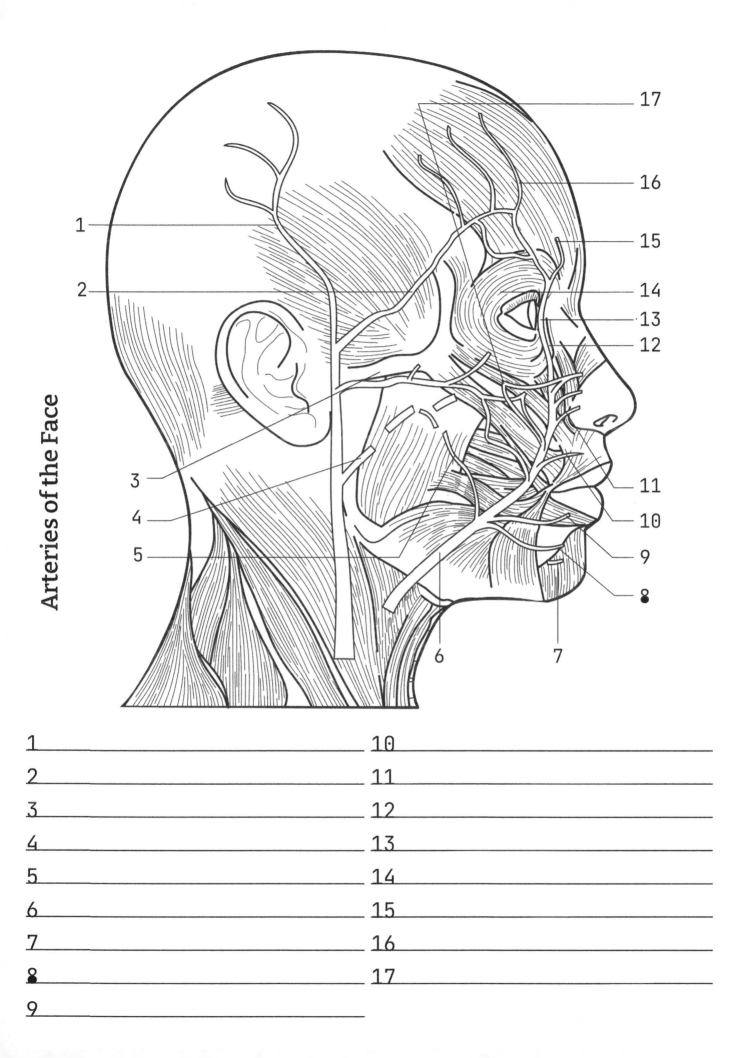

1 _____ 10 _____

2 _____ 11 _____

3 _____ 12 _____

4 _____ 13 _____

5 _____ 14 _____

6 _____ 15 _____

7 _____ 16 _____

8 _____ 17 _____

9 _____

Veins of the Face

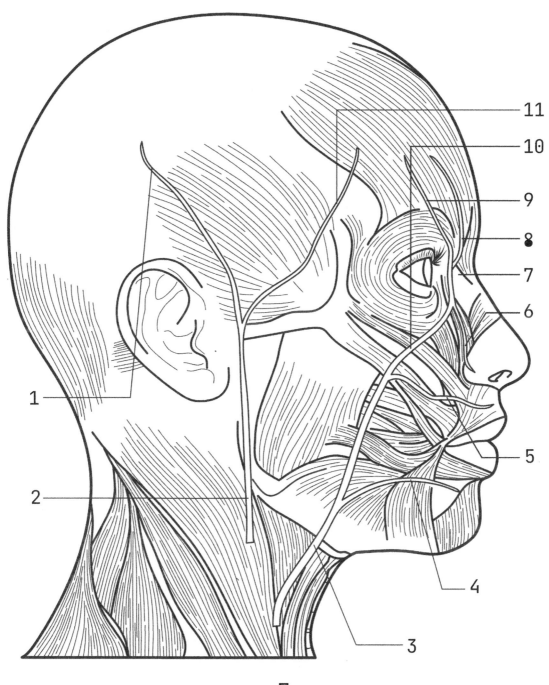

1 _____ 7 _____

2 _____ 8 _____

3 _____ 9 _____

4 _____ 10 _____

5 _____ 11 _____

6 _____

Nerves of the Face

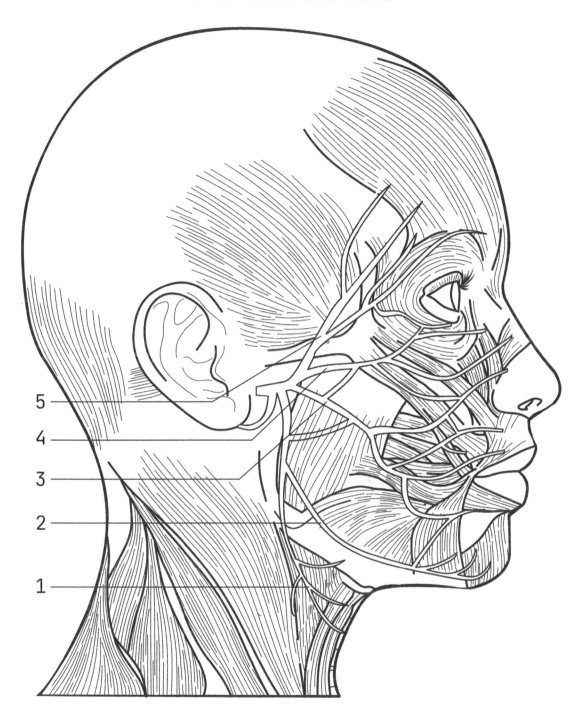

1 _____

2 _____

3 _____

4 _____

5 _____

Trunk of the Facial Nerve

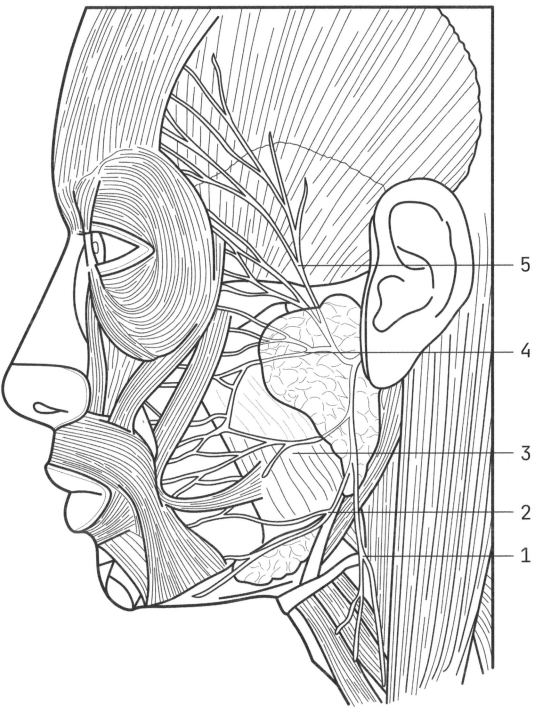

5 _____

4 _____

3 _____

2 _____

1 _____

1 _____

2 _____

3 _____

4 _____

5 _____

Cartilage of the Nose - *Basal View*

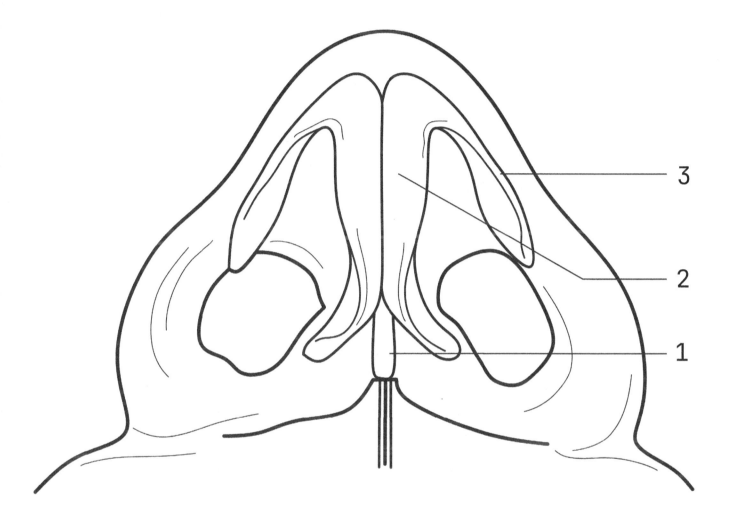

1 _____

2 _____

3 _____

Cartilage of the Nose - Frontal View

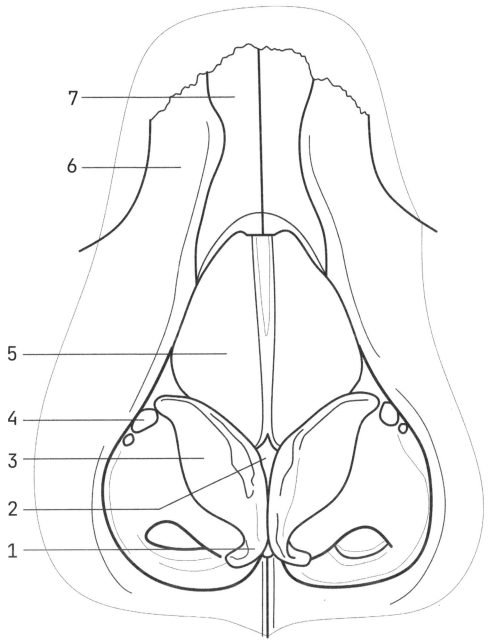

1 _____

2 _____

3 _____

4 _____

5 _____

6 _____

7 _____

Cartilage of the Nose - Oblique View

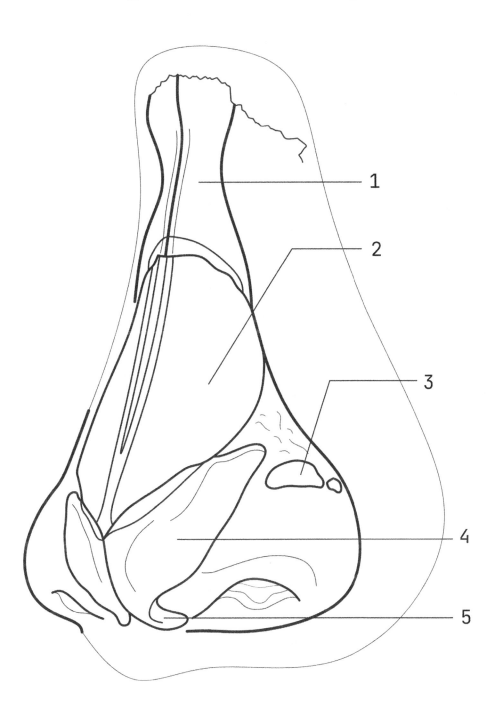

1

2

3

4

5

Deep fat Compartments of the Face

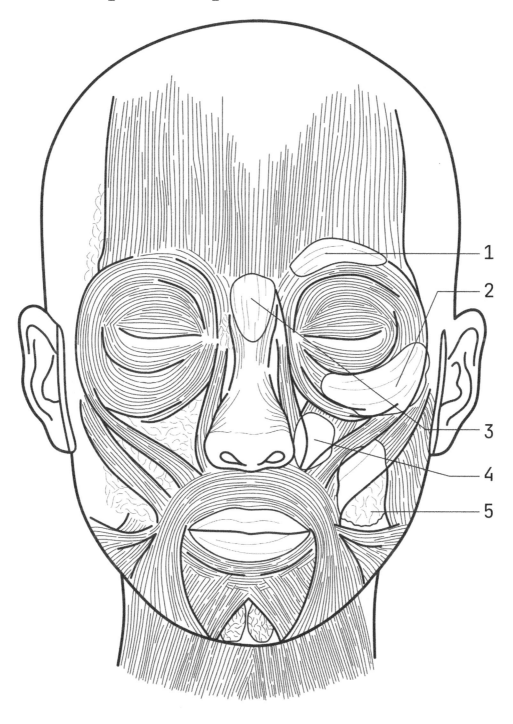

1 _____

2 _____

3 _____

4 _____

5 _____

General Concept About the Course of the Facial Artery

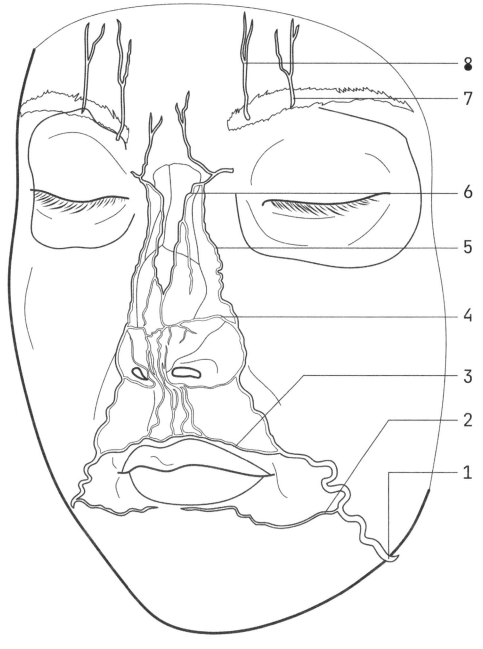

1 _____

2 _____

3 _____

4 _____

5 _____

6 _____

7 _____

8 _____

General Course of the Facial Vein and its Topographic Relationships with the Facial Muscles

1 _____

2 _____

3 _____

4 _____

5 _____

6 _____

7 _____

8 _____

9 _____

10 _____

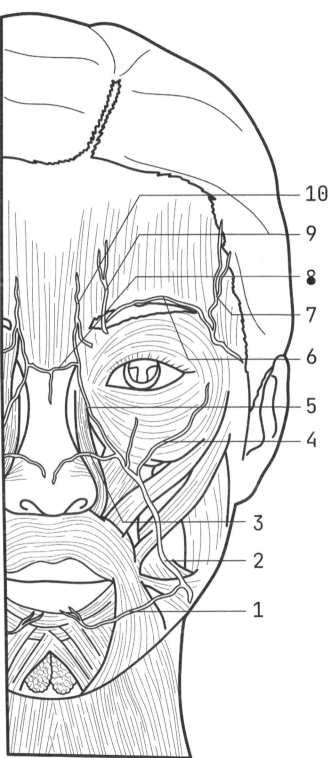

Maxillary Artery and its Branches

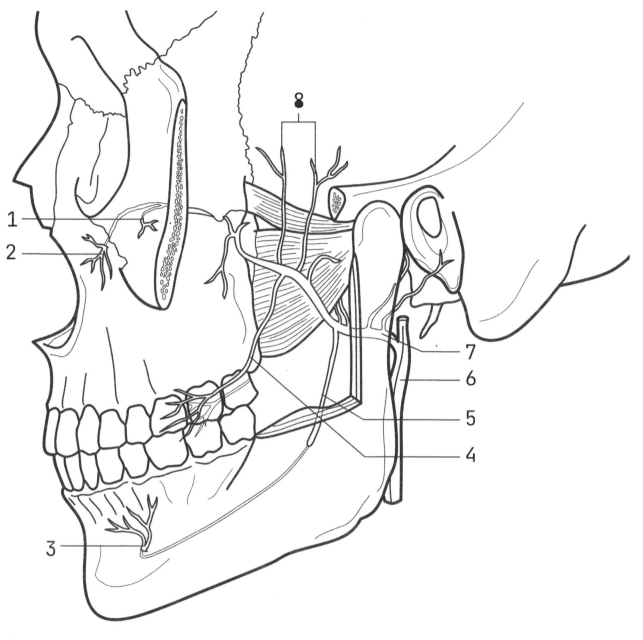

1 _____

2 _____

3 _____

4 _____

5 _____

6 _____

7 _____

8 _____

Nerve Innervations on the Forehead and Temple

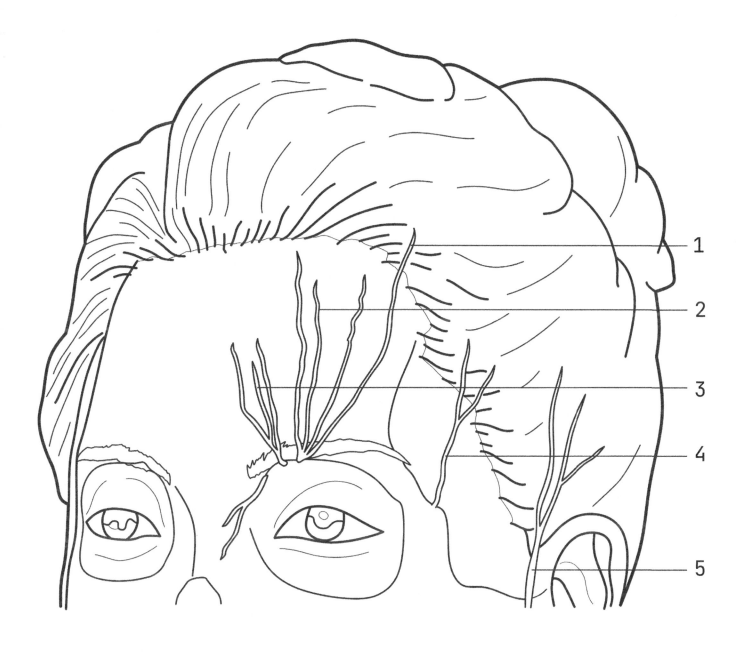

1 _____

2 _____

3 _____

4 _____

5 _____

Superficial Fat and Superficial Muscles of the Face

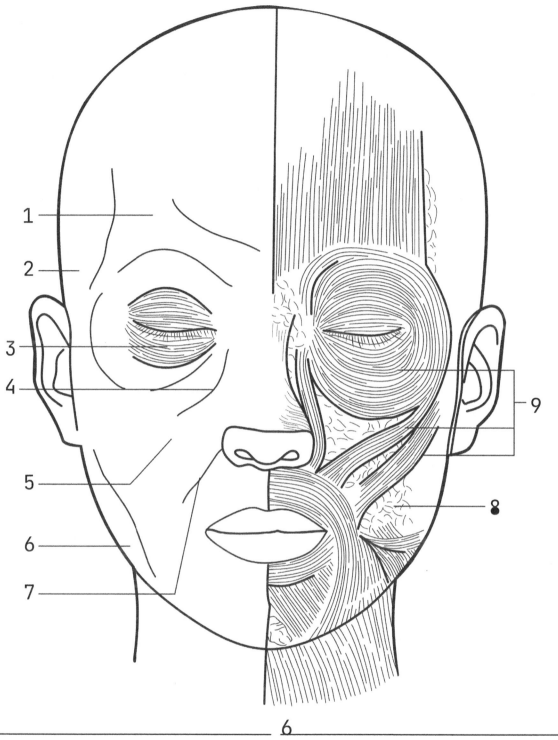

1 _____   6 _____

2 _____   7 _____

3 _____   8 _____

4 _____   9 _____

5 _____

Superficial Musculoaponeurotic System

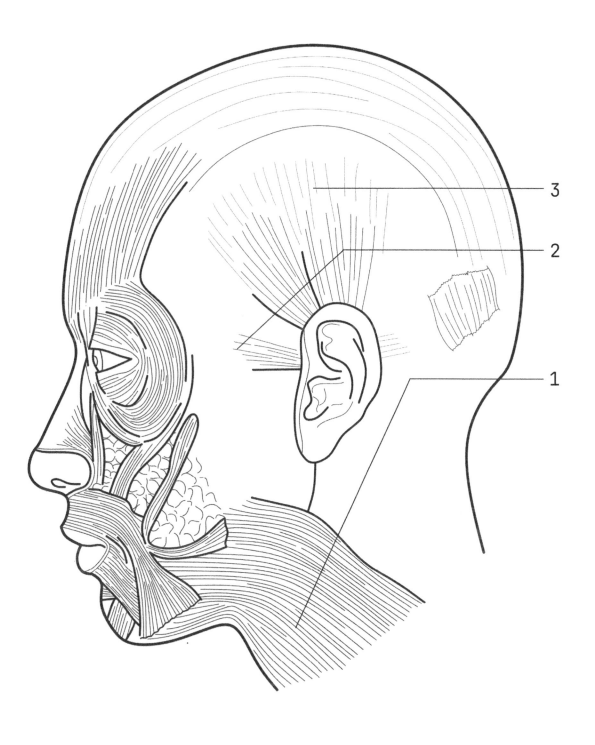

1 _____

2 _____

3 _____

Topographic Anatomy of Peripheral Sensory Nerve Branches of the Head and Neck

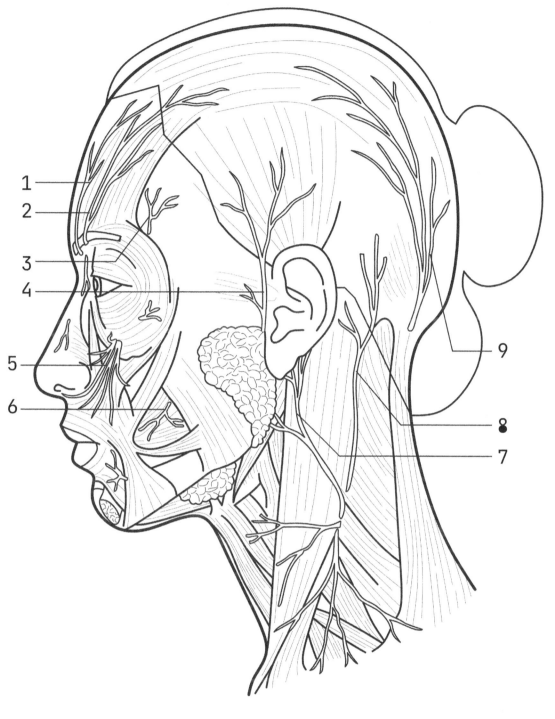

1 _____   6 _____

2 _____   7 _____

3 _____   8 _____

4 _____   9 _____

5 _____

Periorbital Arterial Distribution of the Ophthalmic Artery
(Internal Carotid Arterial System)

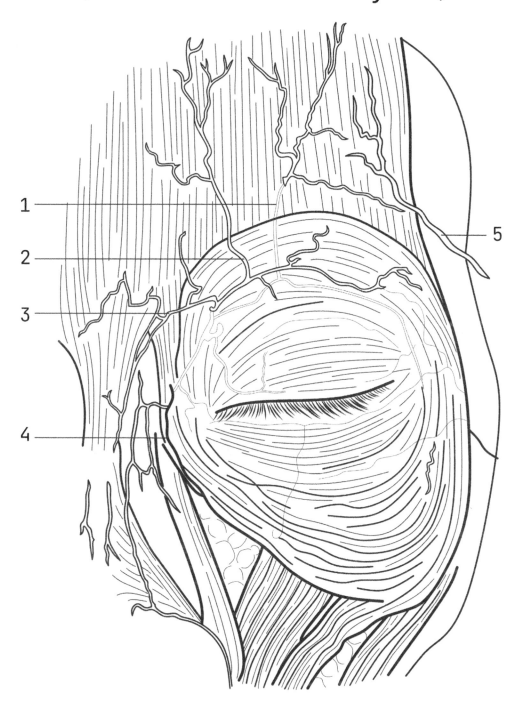

1 _____

2 _____

3 _____

4 _____

5 _____

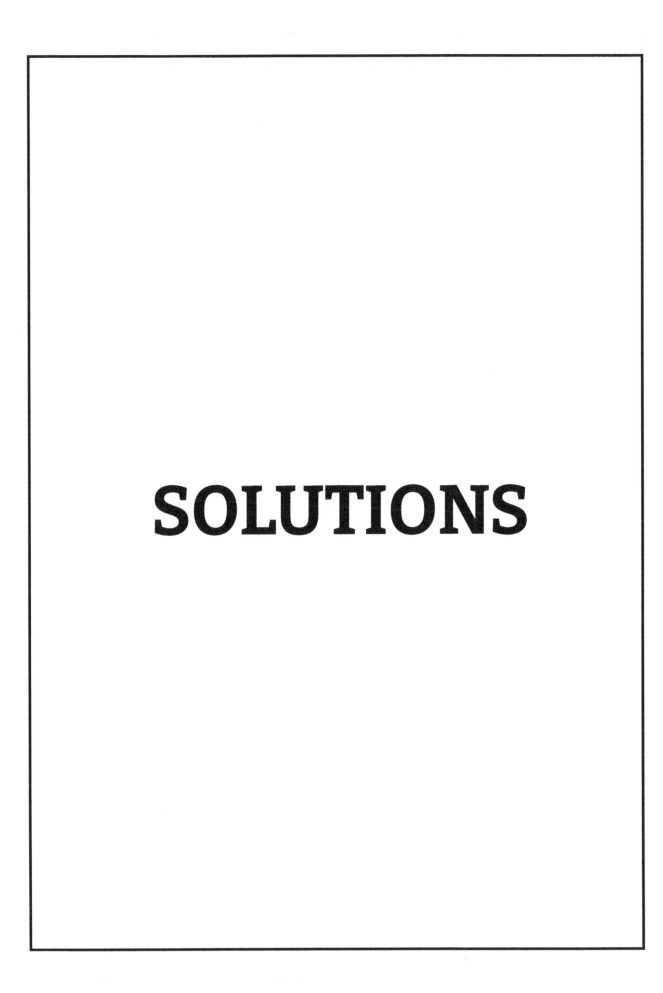

SOLUTIONS

Facial Muscles - *Frontal view*

1. Frontalis m.
2. Orbicularis oculi m.
3. Zygomaticus major m.
4. Zygomaticus minor m.
5. Levator labii superioris m.
6. Risorius m.
7. Depressor anguli oris m.
8. Depressor labii inferioris m.
9. Platysma m.
10. Mentalis m.
11. Orbicularis oris m.
12. Levator anguli oris m.
13. Levator labii superioris alaque nasi m.
14. Depressor supercilii m.
15. Corrugator supercilii m.

Facial Muscles - *Oblique view*

1. Platysma m.
2. Mentalis m.
3. Depressor labii inferioris m.
4. Orbicularis oris m.
5. Depressor anguli oris m.
6. Risorius m.
7. Zygomaticus major m.
8. Zygomaticus minor m.
9. Levator labii superioris m.
10. Levator labii superioris alaque nasi m.
11. Orbicularis oculi m.
12. Nasalis m.
13. Frontalis m.

Facial Muscles - *Lateral view*

1. Platysma m.
2. Risorius m.
3. Mentalis m.
4. Depressor anguli oris m.
5. Deressor labii inferioris m.
6. Orbicularis oris m.
7. Zygomaticus major m.
8. Zygomaticus minor m.
9. Levator labii superioris m.
10. Nasalis m.
11. labii superioris alaque nasi m.
12. Orbicularis oculi m.
13. Frontalis m.

Muscles of the lower face

1. Depressor anguli oris
2. Mentalis
3. Orbicularis oris
4. Modiolus
5. Platysma
6. Depressor labii inferioris
7. sternal part of the sternocleidomastoid muscle
8. clavicular part of the sternocleidomastoid muscle

Muscles of the Midface

1. Zygomaticus major
2. Buccinator
3. Risorius
4. Levator anguli oris (deep to all others except buccinator)

5. Zygomaticus minor

6. Nasalis

7. Nasal part of the levator labii superioris alaeque nasi

8. Labial part of levator labii superioris alaeque nasi

Muscles of the Upper Face

1. Corrugator supercilii (deep to orbicularis oculi)

2. Procerus

3. Depressor supercilii

4. Orbicularis oculi

5. Frontalis

Perinasal Muscles

1. Nasalis m. (alar part)

2. Depressor septi m.

3. levator labii superioris alaque nasi m.

4. Nasalis m. (transverse part)

5. Orbicularis oculi m.

6. Procerus m.

Perioral Muscles

1. Zygomaticus major m.

2. Zygomaticus minor m.

3. Risorius m.

4. Levator labii superioris m.

5. Depressor anguli oris m.

6. Depressor labii inferioris m.

7. Platysma m.

8. Mentalis m.

9. Orbicularis oris m.

10. Levator labii superioris alaque nasi m.

11. Levator anguli oris m.

Perioral Muscles

1. Depressor anguli oris m.

2. Risorius m.

3. Zygomaticus major m.

4. Orbicularis oris m.

5. Levator anguli oris m.

Anatomical Layers of the Face - *Basic five layers of the Face*

1. Skin

2. Subcutaneous layer

3. Facial mm. & superficial musculoaponeurotic system (SMAS)

4. Retaining ligament and space

5. Periosteum and deep fascia

Anatomical Layers of the Forehead and Glabella

1. Periosteum

2. Frontal bone

3. Loose connective tissue

4. Frontalis m. and galea aponeurosis

5. Subcutaneous layer

6. Skin

Arteries of the Face

1. Posterior branch of superficial temporal artery
2. Anterior branch of superficial temporal artery
3. Transverse facial
4. Maxillary
5. Lingual
6. Facial
7. Mental
8. Horizontal Mental
9. Inferior labial
10. Superior labial
11. Alar branch of facial artery
12. Angular
13. Dorsal nasal
14. Infratrochlear
15. Supratrochlear
16. Supraorbital artery
17. Infraorbital

Veins of the face

1. Lingual
2. Supratrochlear
3. Dorsal nasal
4. Supraorbital artery
5. Angular
6. Superior labial
7. Inferior labial
8. Facial
9. Horizontal mental
10. Alar branch of facial artery
11. Transverse facial

Nerves of the Face

1. cervical

2. marginal mandibular

3. buccal

4. Zygomatic

5. temporal

Trunk of the Facial Nerve

1. Cervical br.

2. Marginal mandibular br.

3. Buccal br.

4. Zygomatic br.

5. Temporal br.

Cartilage of the Nose - Basal View

1. Septal nasal cartilage

2. Greater alar cartilage (medial crus)

3. Greater alar cartilage (lateral crus)

Cartilage of the Nose - Frontal View

1. Greater alar cartilage (medial crus)

2. Septal nasal cartilage

3. Greater alar cartilage (lateral crus)

4. Lesser alar cartilage

5. Lateral nasal cartilage

6. Frontal process of maxilla

7. Nasal bone

Cartilage of the Nose - Oblique View

1. Nasal bone
2. Lateral nasal cartilage
3. Lesser alar cartilage
4. Greater alar cartilage (lateral crus)
5. Greater alar cartilage (medial crus)

Deep Fat Compartments of the Face

1. Retro-orbicularis oculi fat (ROOF)
2. Suborbicularis oculi fat (SOOF)
3. Subprocerus galeal fat
4. Deep medial cheek fat
5. Buccal fat pad

General Concept About the Course of the Facial Artery

1. Facial a.
2. Inferior alar br.
3. Superior labial a.
4. Lateral nasal a.
5. Angular a.
6. Dorsal nasal a.
7. Supraorbital a.
8. Supratrochlear a.

General Course of the Facial Vein and its Topographic Relationships with the Facial Muscles

1. Facial a.
2. Inferior alar br.
3. Superior labial a.

4. Lateral nasal a.

5. Angular a.

6. Dorsal nasal a.

7. Supraorbital a.

8. Supratrochlear a.

Nerve Innervations on the Forehead and Temple

1. Deep br. of supraorbital n.

2. Supraorbital n.

3. Supratrochlear n.

4. Zygomaticotemporal n.

5. Auriculotemporal n.

Superficial fat and Superficial Muscles of the Face

1. Forehead fat compartment

2. Lateral orbital fat compartment

3. Palpebral portion of orbicularis oculi m.

4. Medial muscular band

5. Malar fat compartment

6. Prejowl fat compartment

7. Nasolabial fat compartment

8. Buccal fat pad

9. Retaining ligaments

Superficial musculoaponeurotic system (SMAS)

1. Platysma m.

2. SMAS

3. Temporoparietal fascia

Topographic Anatomy of Peripheral Sensory Nerve Branches of the Head and Neck

1. Supratrochlear n.
2. Supraorbital n.
3. Zygomaticotemporal n.
4. Auriculotemporal n.
5. Infraorbital n.
6. Buccal n.
7. Great auricular n.
8. Lesser occipital n.
9. Greater occipital n.

Periorbital Arterial Distribution of the Ophthalmic Artery (Internal Carotid Arterial System)

1. Supraorbital a.
2. Supratrochlear a.
3. Dorsal nasal a.
4. Angular a.
5. Superficial temporal a.

Made in the USA
Monee, IL
13 August 2023

40933526R10037